MY BODY AND ME

My Beating Heart

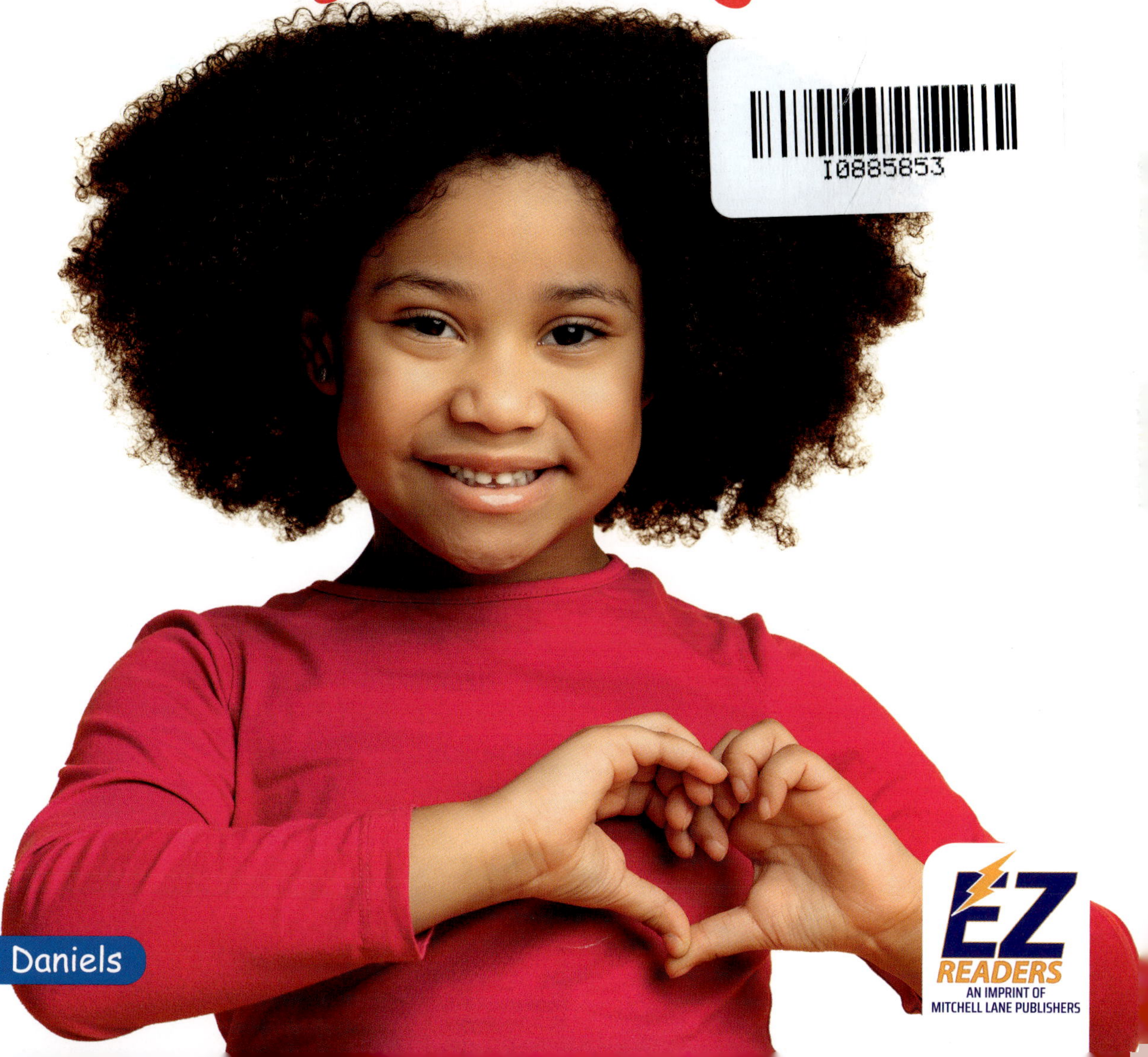

Rachel Daniels

EZ READERS
AN IMPRINT OF
MITCHELL LANE PUBLISHERS

CREATING YOUNG NONFICTION READERS

EZ Readers offer nonfiction for beginning readers in PreK through first grade, using simple language, clear illustrations, and engaging facts to build vocabulary and confidence.

TIPS FOR READING NONFICTION WITH BEGINNING READERS

Talk about Nonfiction

Begin by explaining that nonfiction books give us information that is true. The book will be organized around a specific topic or idea, and we may learn new facts through reading.

Look at the Parts

Most nonfiction books have helpful features. Our *EZ Readers* include color photographs and graphic aids, a table of contents, a glossary, and an index. Share the purpose of these features with your reader.

Color Photos and Graphic Aids

A lot of information can be found by "reading" photos, charts, maps, and other graphic aids found within nonfiction texts. Help your reader learn more about the different ways information can be displayed.

Table of Contents

Located at the front of the book, this list shows the big ideas within the text and the page numbers where they can be found.

Glossary

Located at the back of the book, the glossary defines key words and phrases that are related to the topic. These words and phrases can be found in the text in colored type.

Index

Located at the back of the book, an index is an alphabetical list of topics and the page numbers where they can be found.

With a little help and guidance about reading nonfiction, you can feel good about introducing a young reader to the world of *EZ Readers* nonfiction books.

EZ Readers is an imprint of:

Mitchell Lane
PUBLISHERS

2001 SW 31st Avenue
Hallandale, FL 33009
mitchelllanepub.com

First Edition, 2026.

Author: Rachel Daniels
Editor: Morgan Brody

Author: Kerrily Sapet
Editor: Morgan Brody

ISBN 979-8-89260-824-4 (library binding)
ISBN 979-8-90145-030-7 (paperback)
ISBN 979-8-89260-835-0 (ebook)

LC record available at https://lccn.loc.gov/2025950825

Photo credits: Shutterstock, Alex Konon, cover, 1, 2, 3, 5, 6, 10, 17, 21; yusuf_demirci, cover, 1; Prostock-studio, cover, 1; Krakenimages.com, 4, 22; Tama2u, 7; dezign56, 7, 22; Prostock-studio, 8–9; Samuel Borges Photography, 11; alexei_tm, 12; hot4Sell, 14–15, 22; Prostock-studio, 16, 22; shutt2016, 18–19; Ekaterina Markelova, 20

Table of Contents

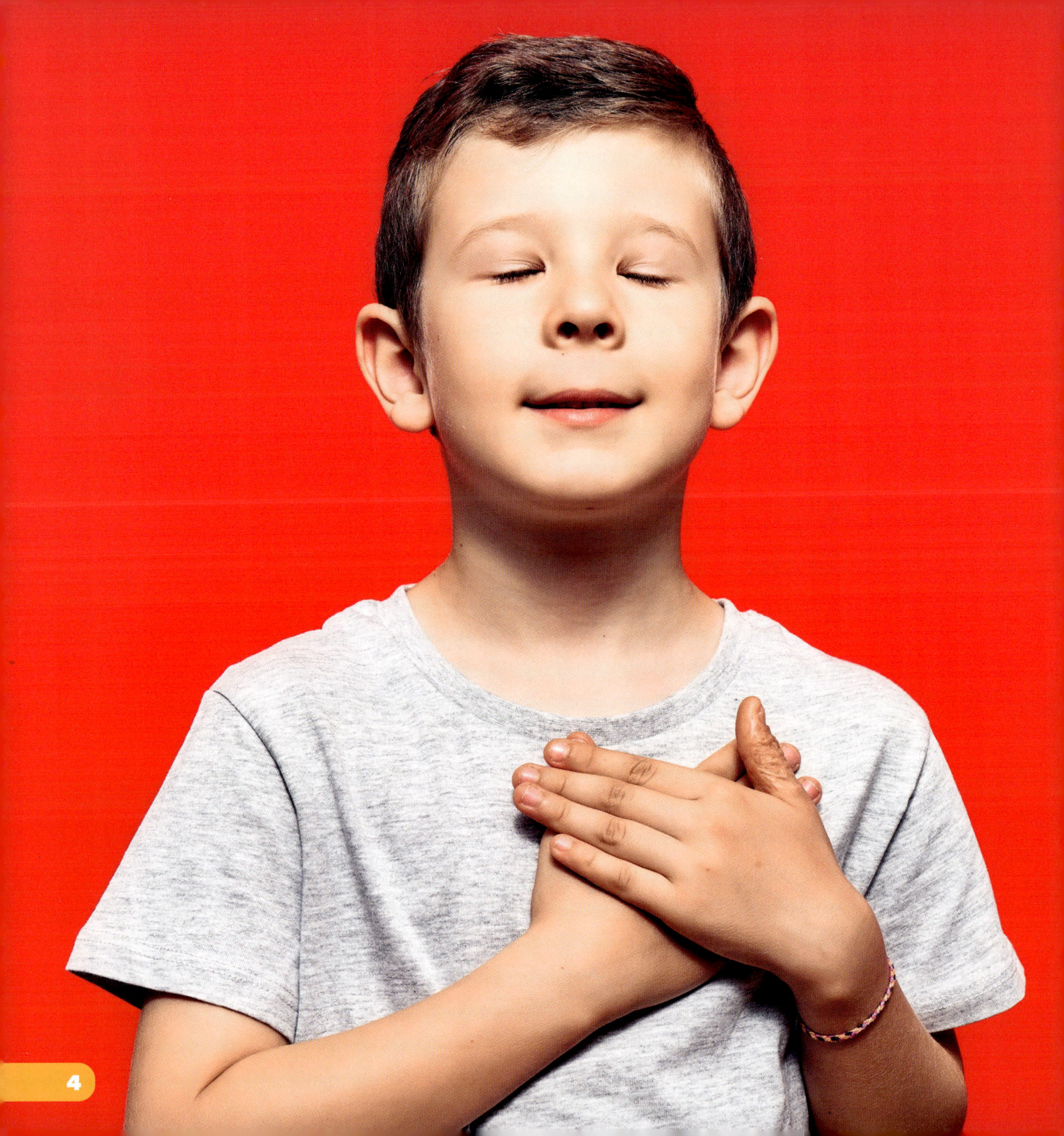

Feel Your Heart

Put your hand on your **chest**.

Do you feel it?

Thump-thump. Thump-thump.

That is your **heart**!

Where Is It?

Your heart is in your chest.

It sits a little to the left.

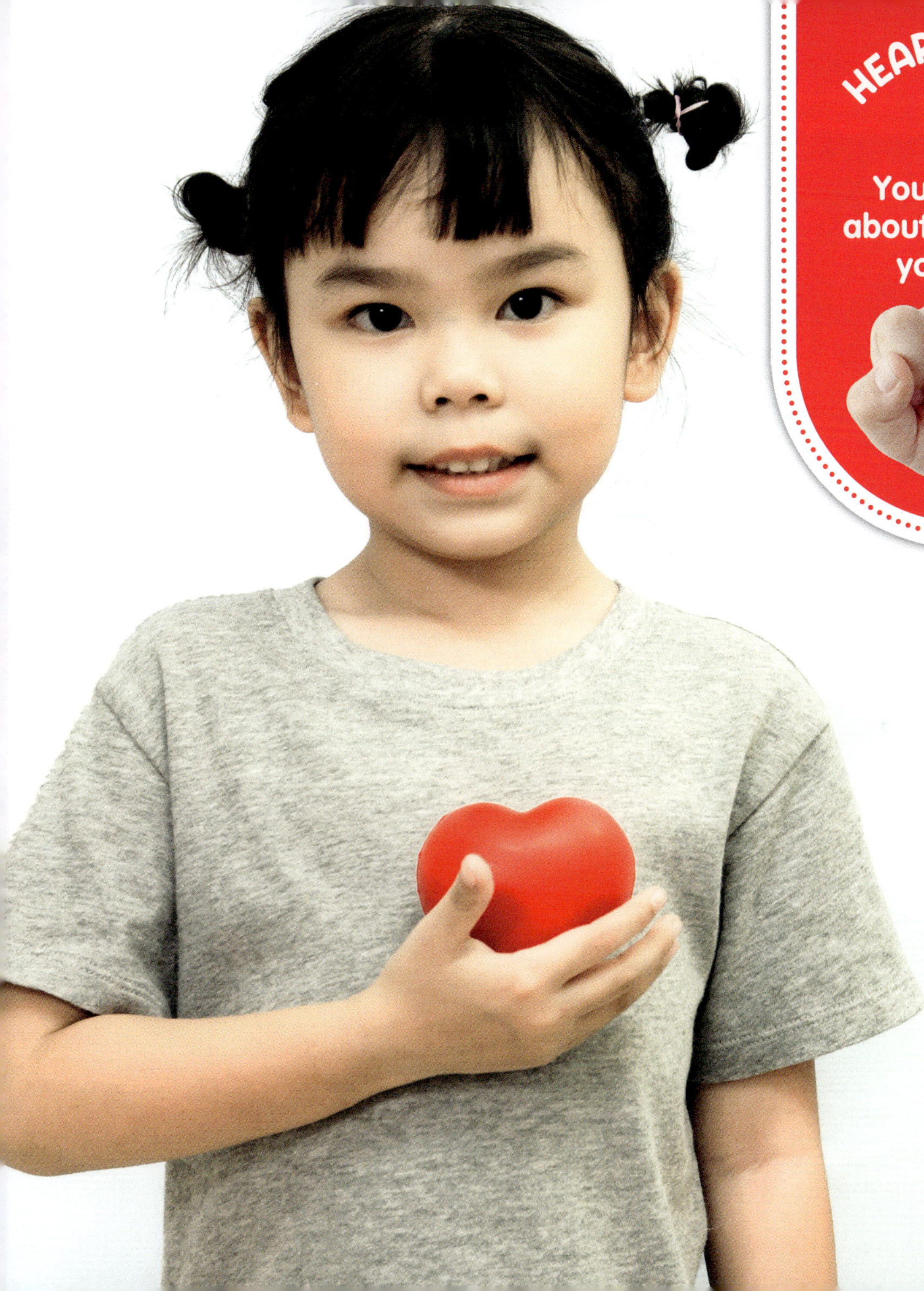

HEART SMART

Your heart is about the size of your **fist**.

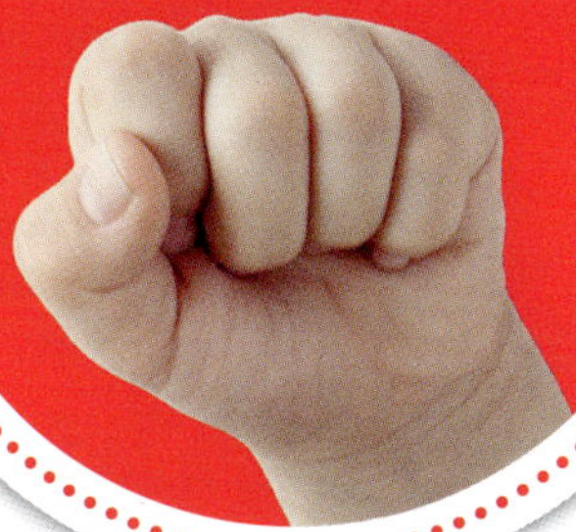

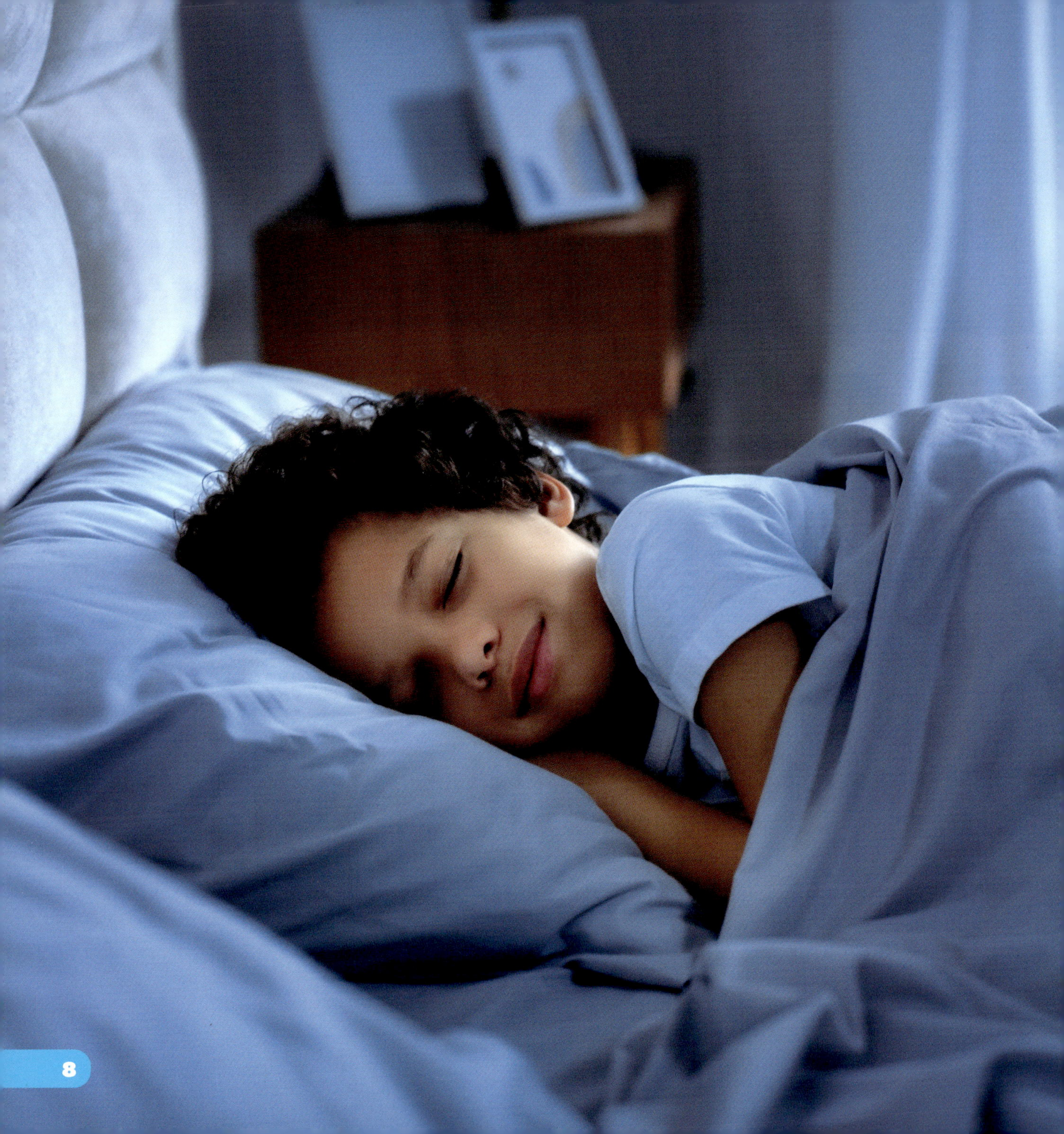

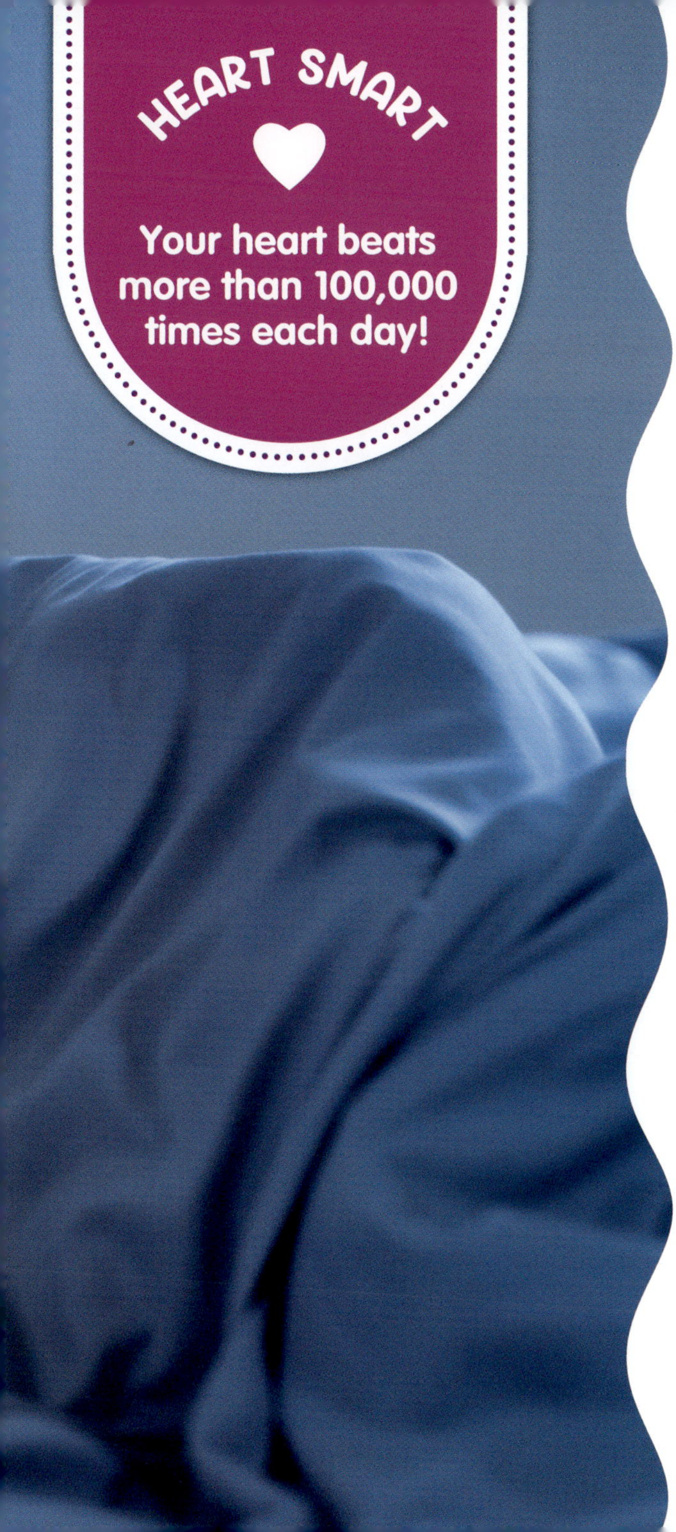
HEART SMART
Your heart beats more than 100,000 times each day!

Thump-thump.
Thump-thump.

That is the sound of your heart.

It **beats** all day and night.

All the Time

Your heart works when you eat.

It works when you read.

It works when you sleep.

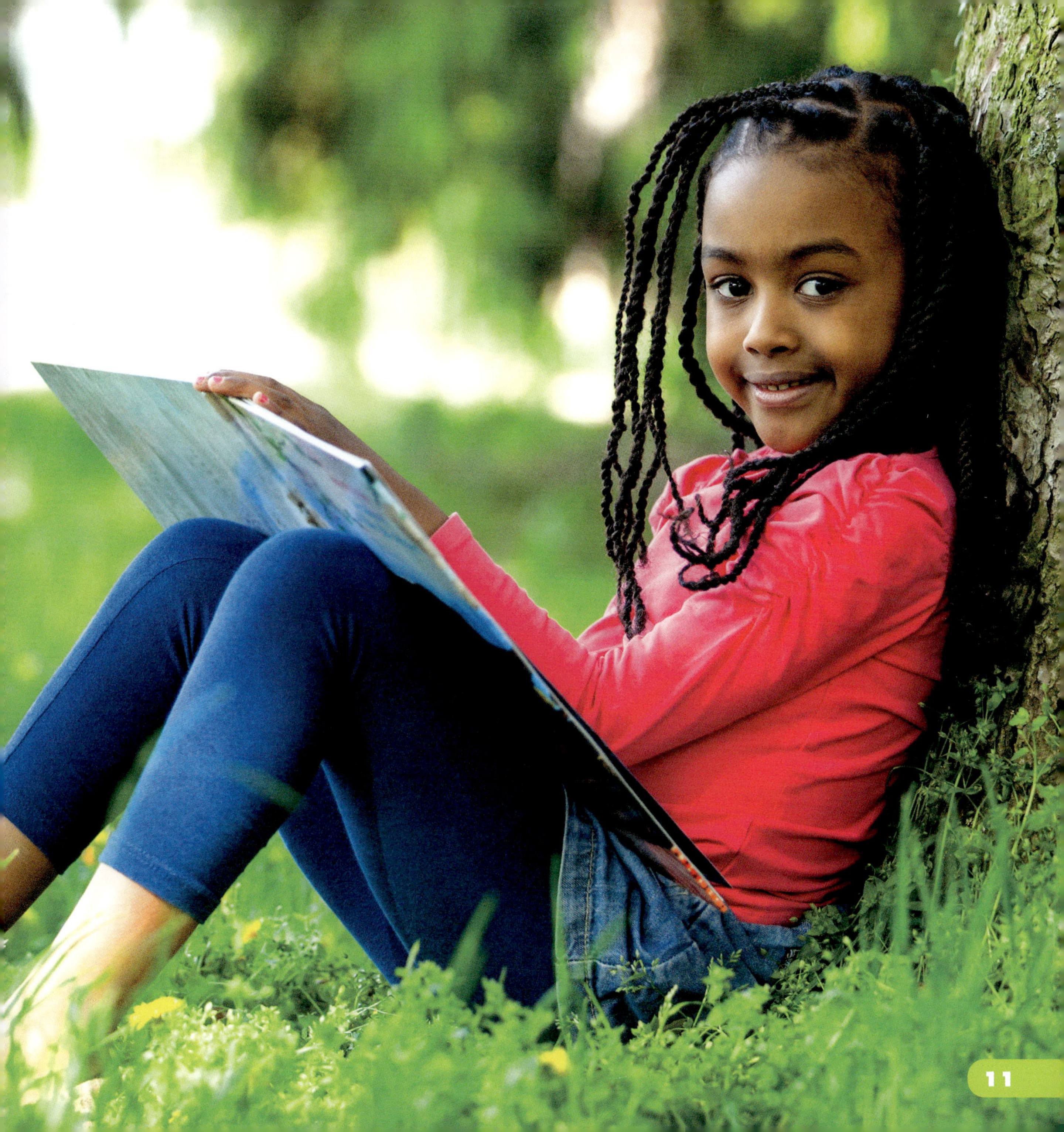

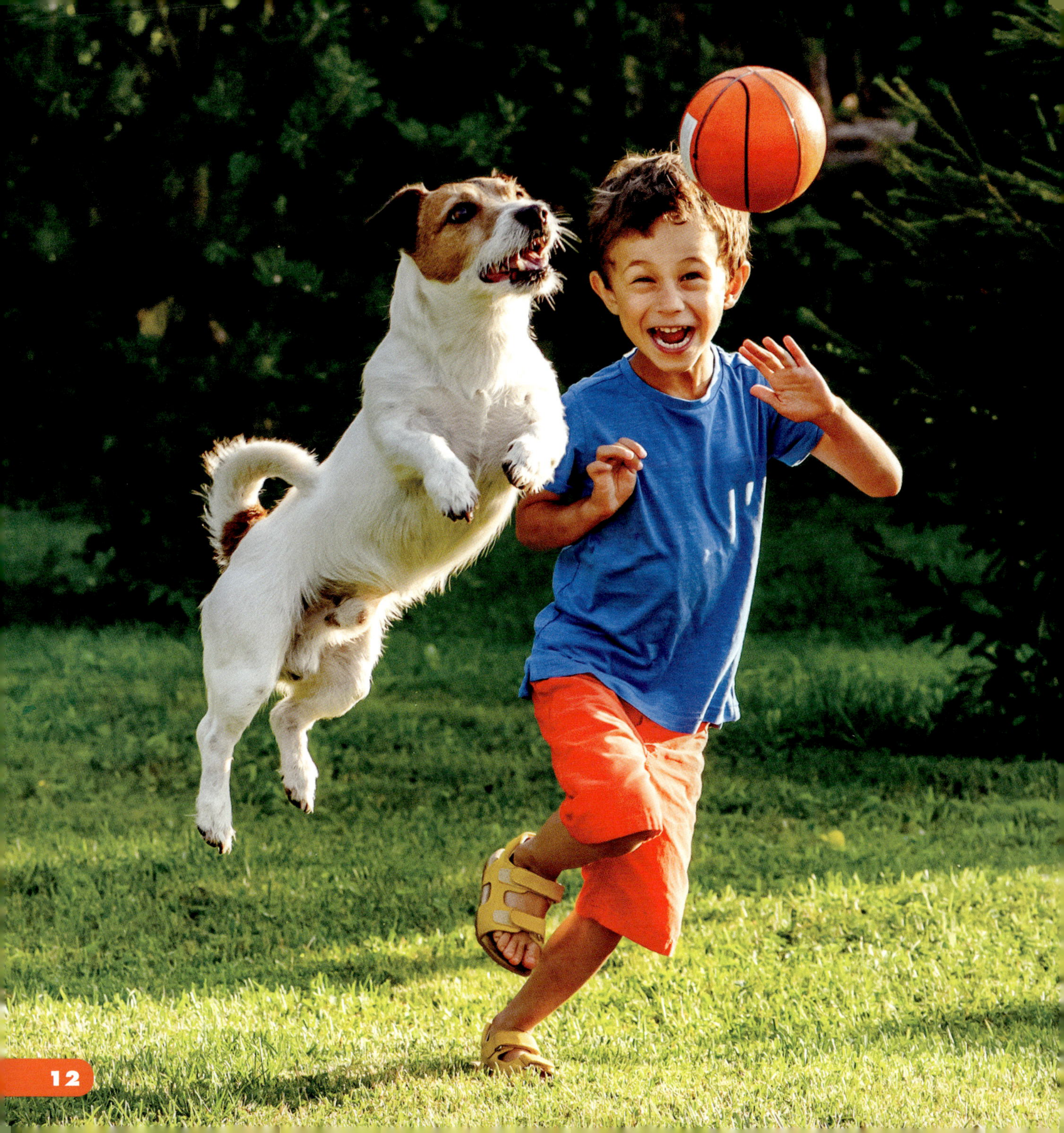

Your heart beats fast when you run.
Your heart beats slow when you rest.

Blood goes out.

Blood comes back.

It moves all day long.

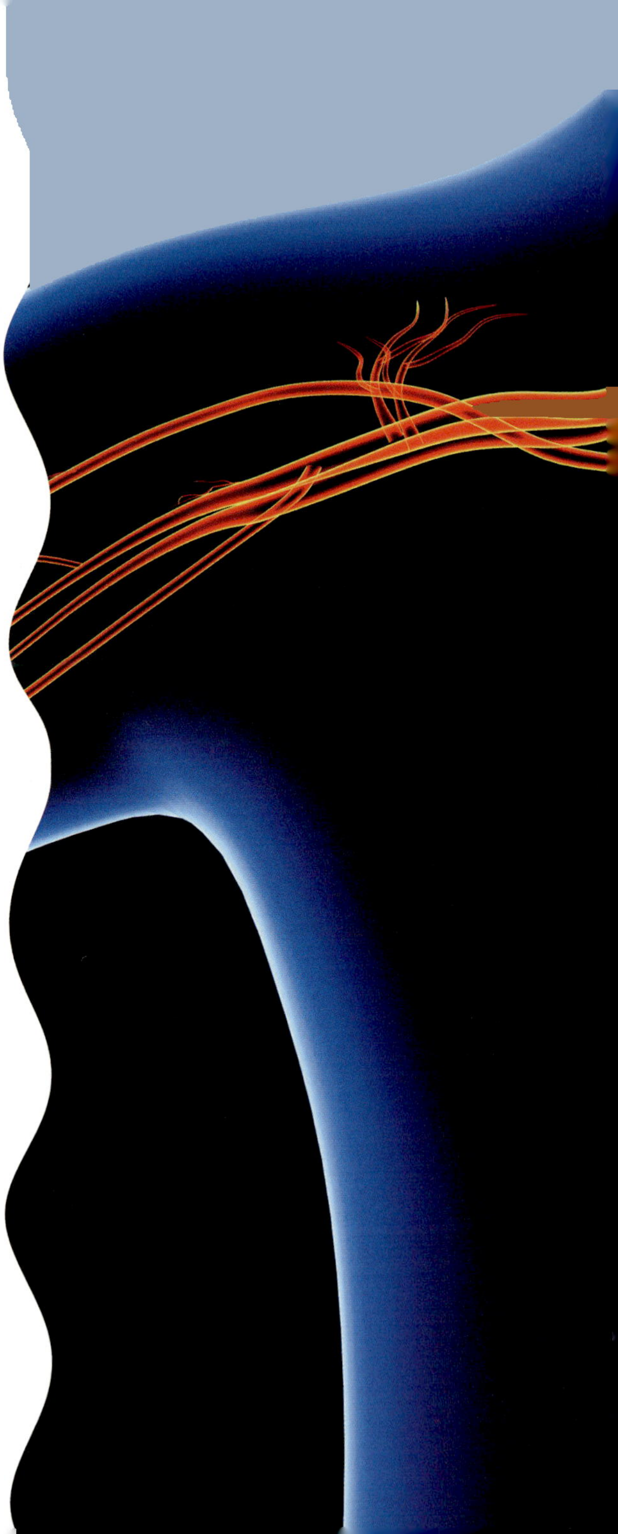

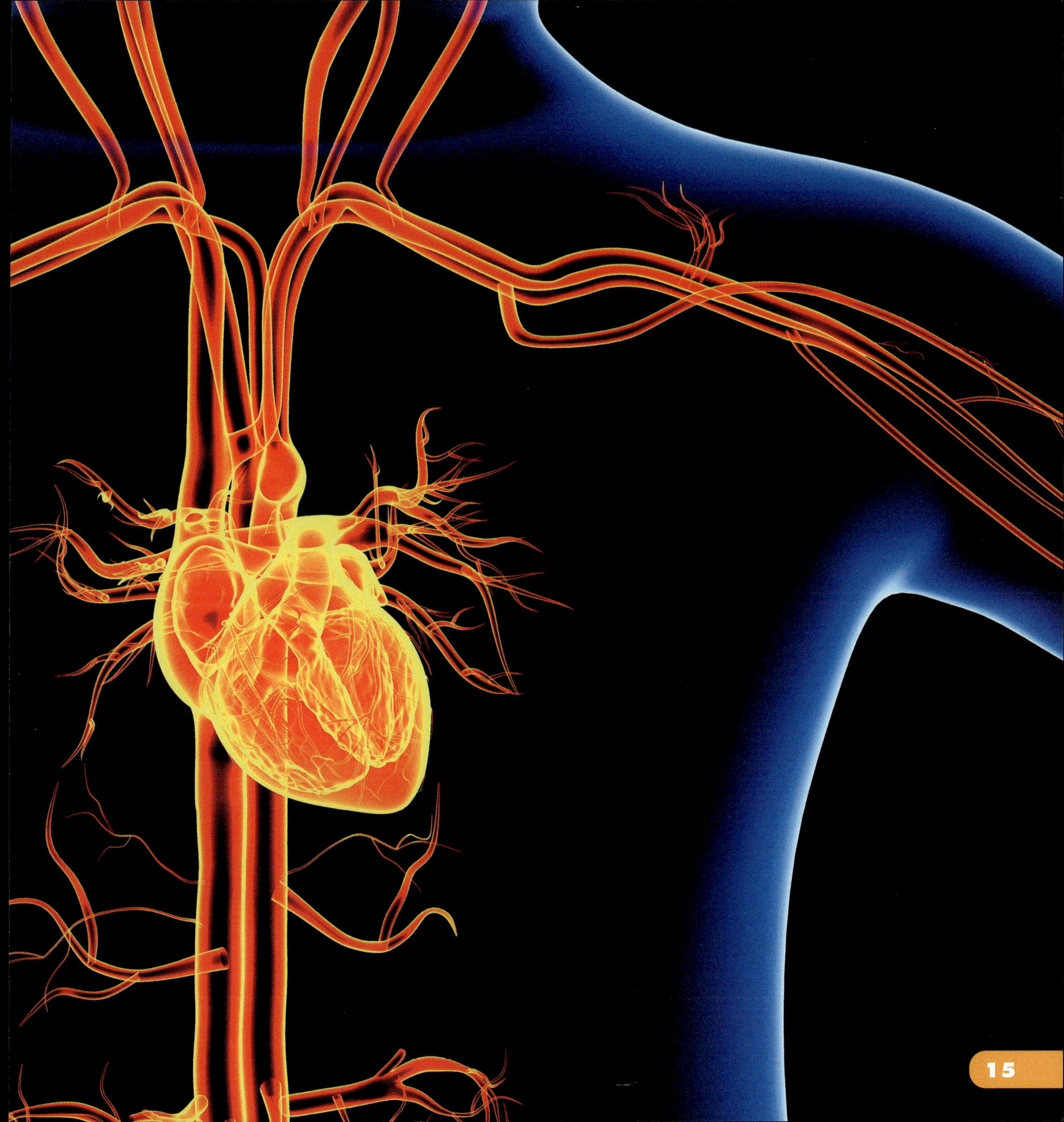

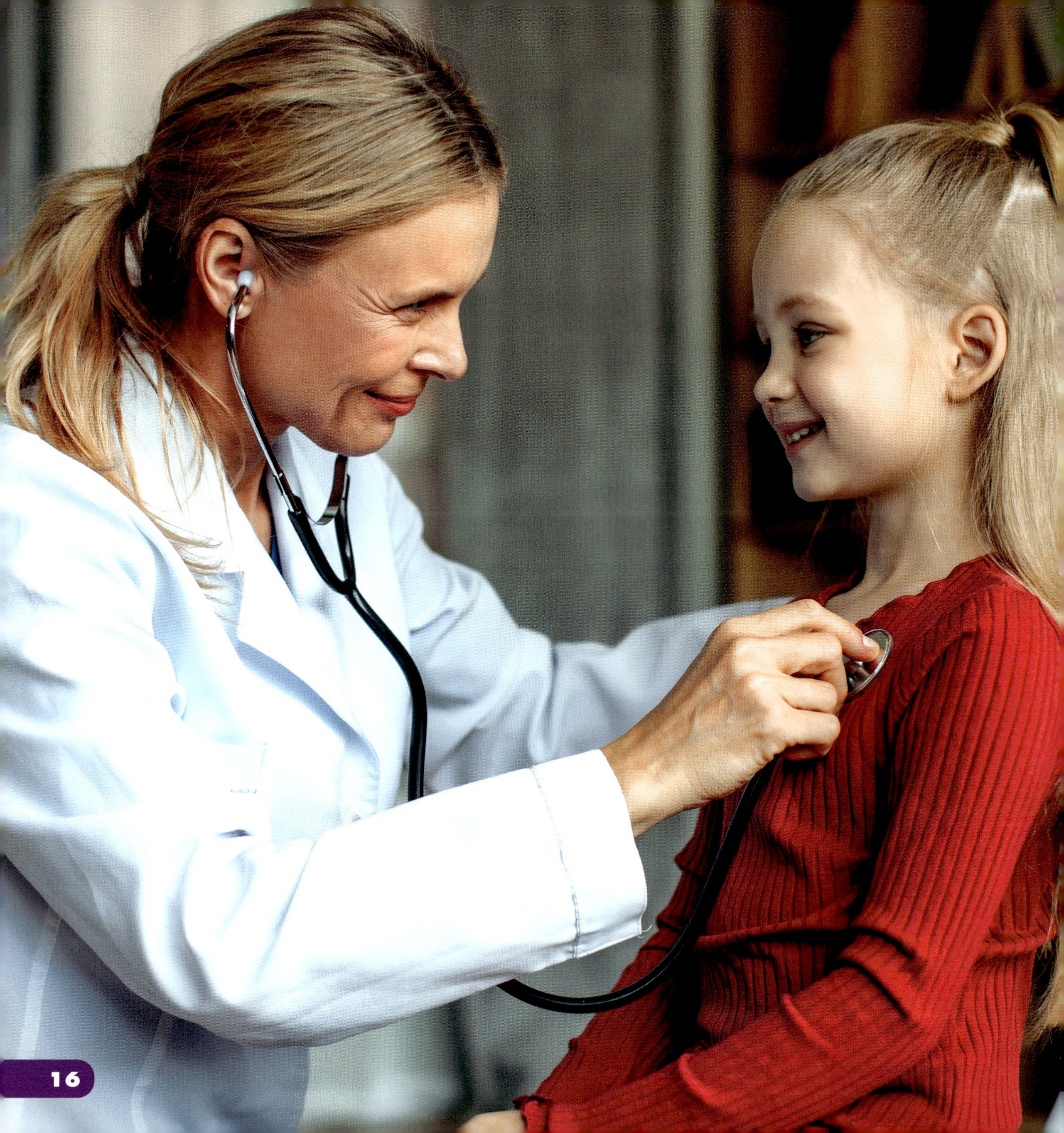

Listen

Doctors use a **stethoscope**.

They listen to your heart.

Thump-thump. Thump-thump.

Your heart started beating before you were born.

It will beat your whole life.

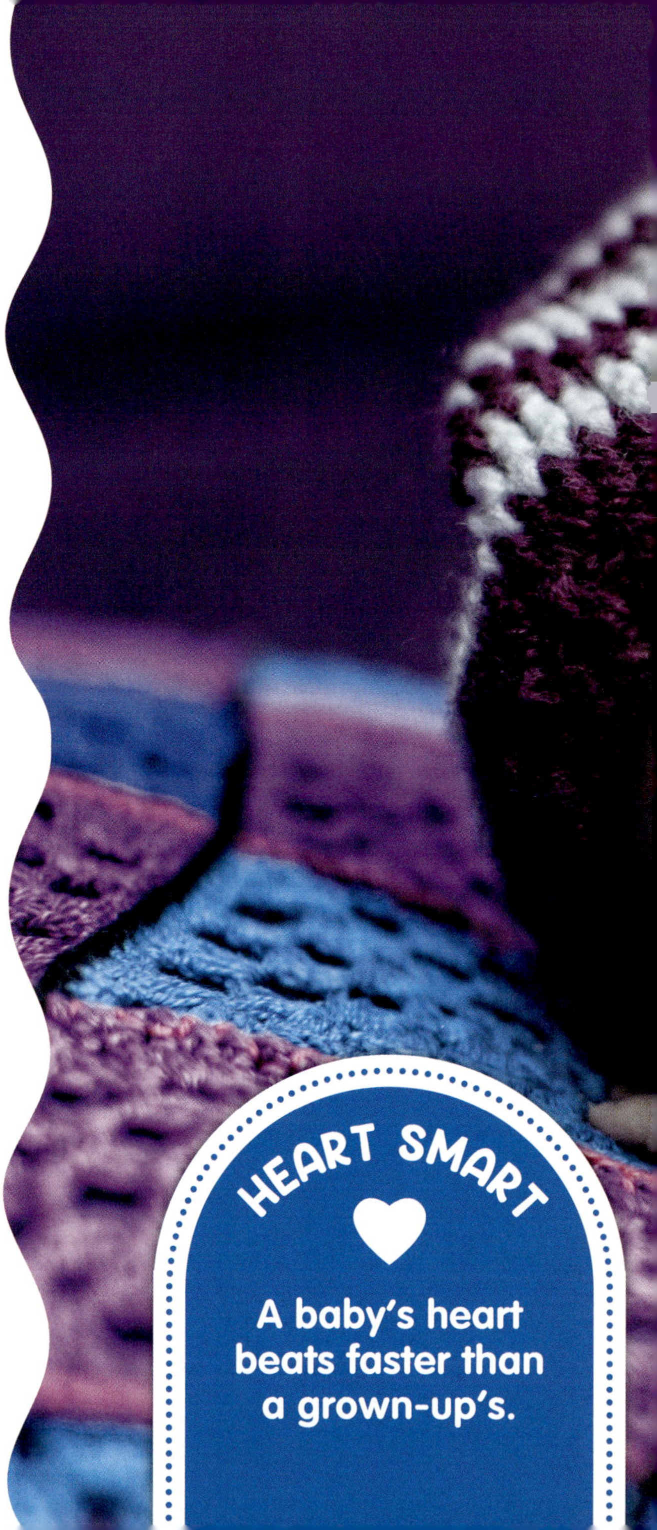

HEART SMART

A baby's heart beats faster than a grown-up's.

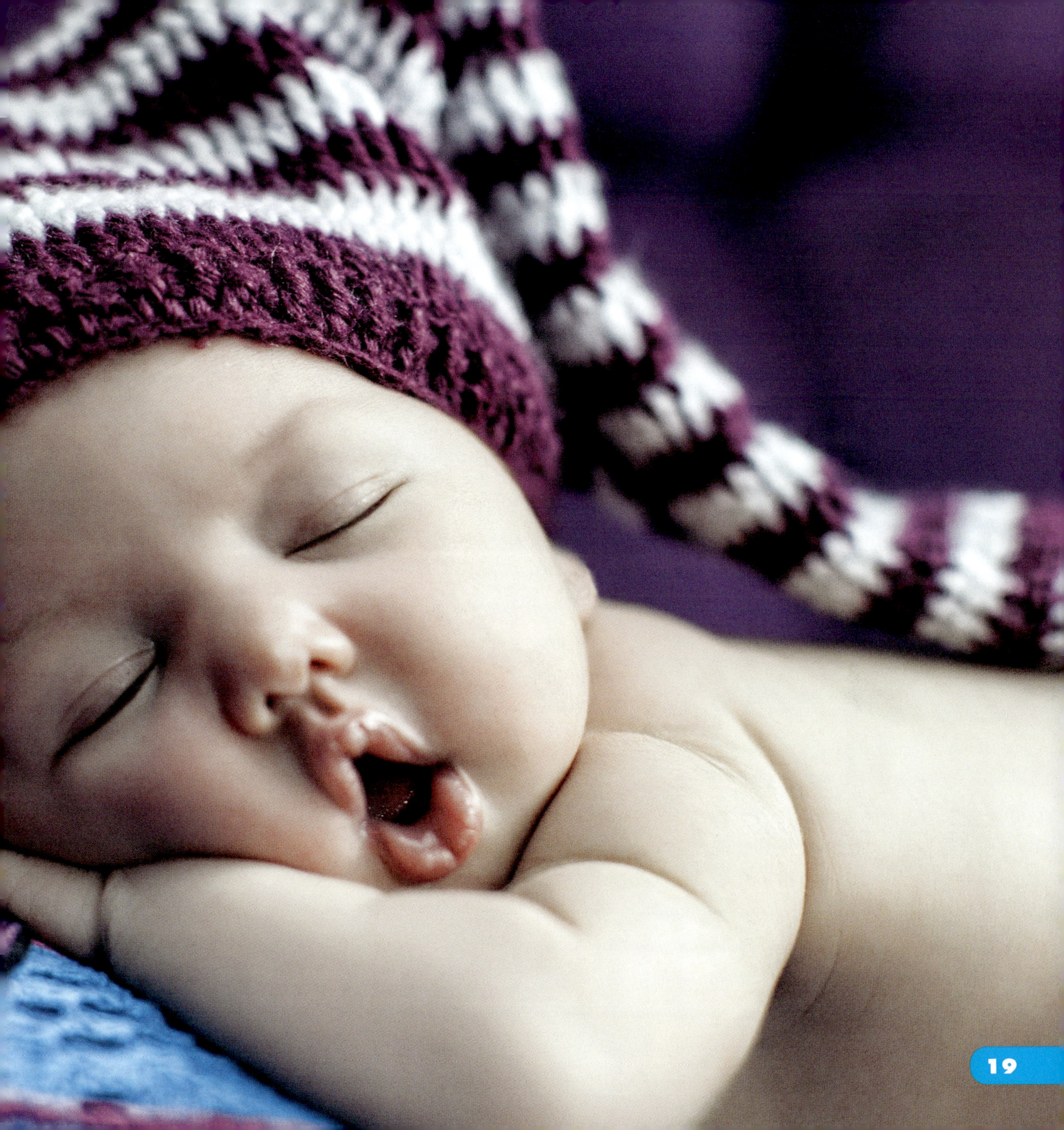

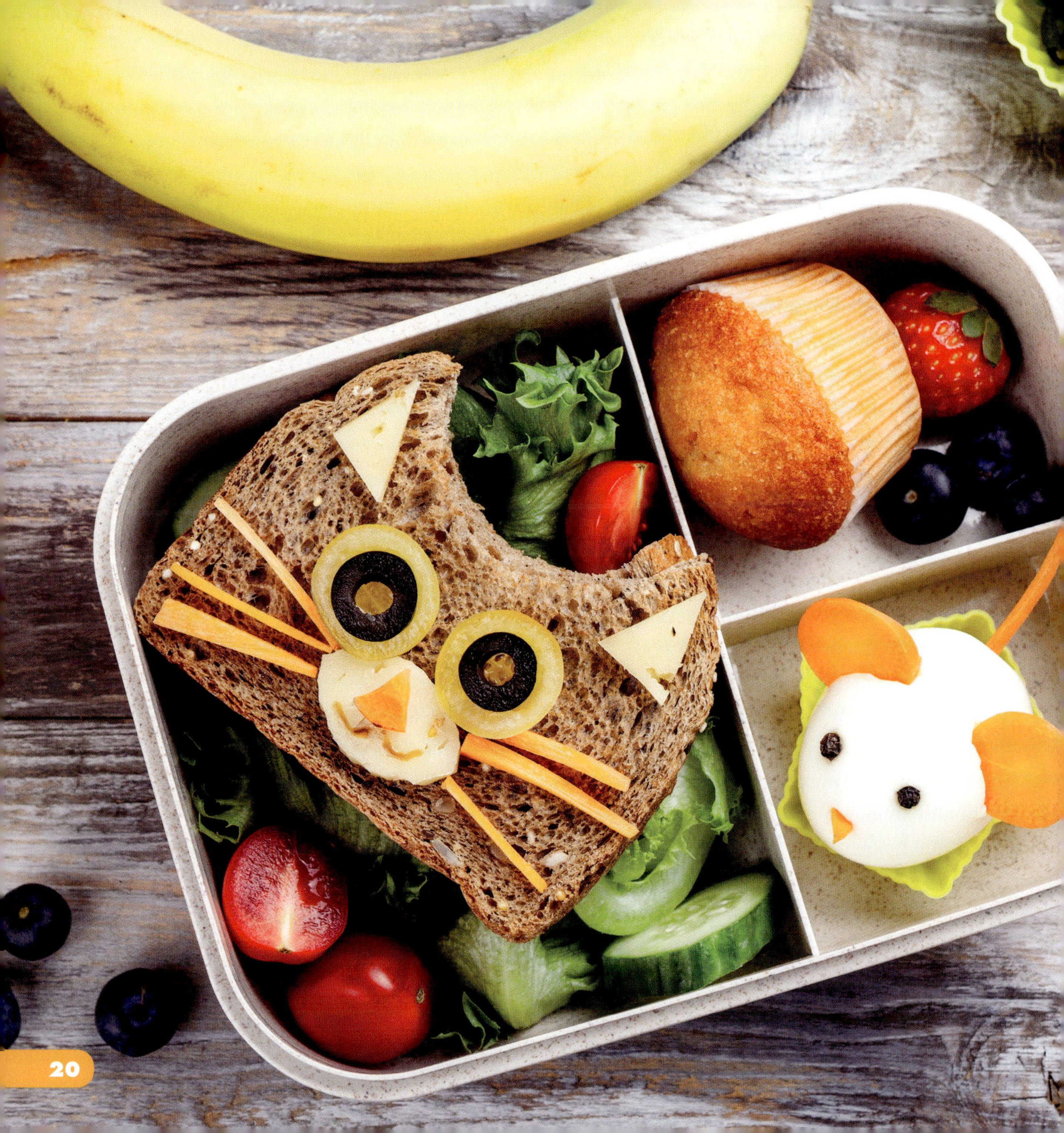

Keep It Strong

Eat good food.

Run, jump, and play.

Take care of your heart!

Glossary

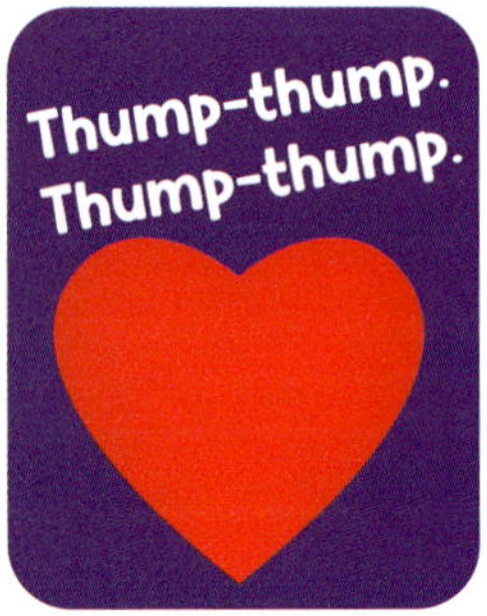

beat (bēet) the sound your heart makes when it pumps blood

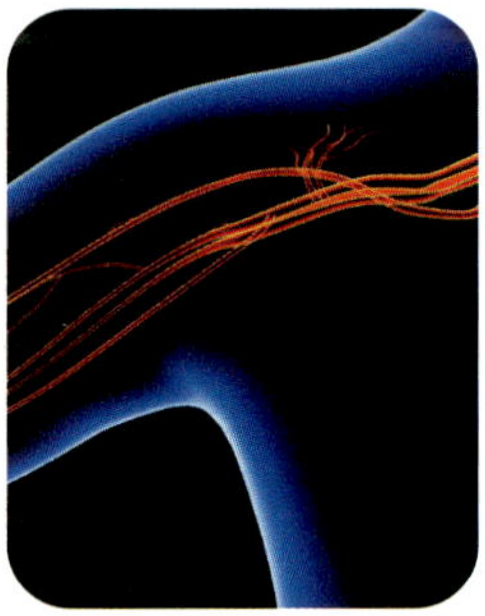

blood (bluhd) the red liquid that moves through your body carrying food and oxygen

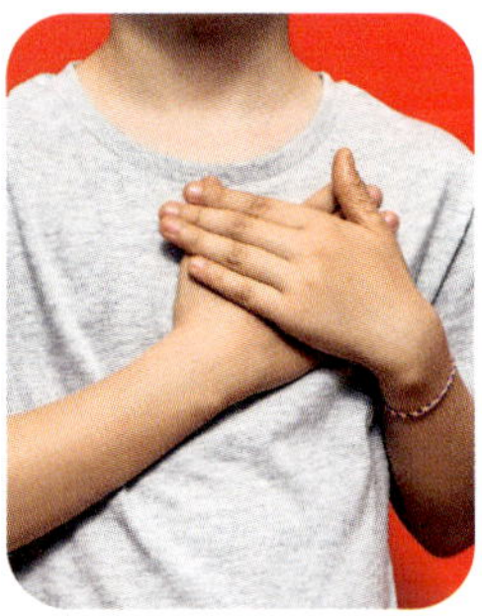

chest (chest) the part of your body where your heart is

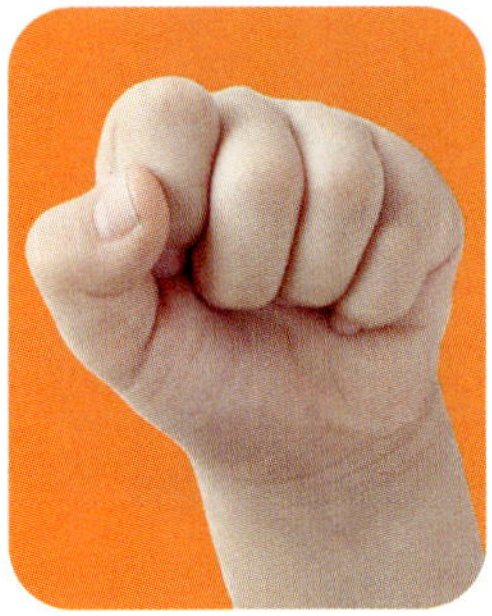

fist (fist) your hand when you make a tight ball

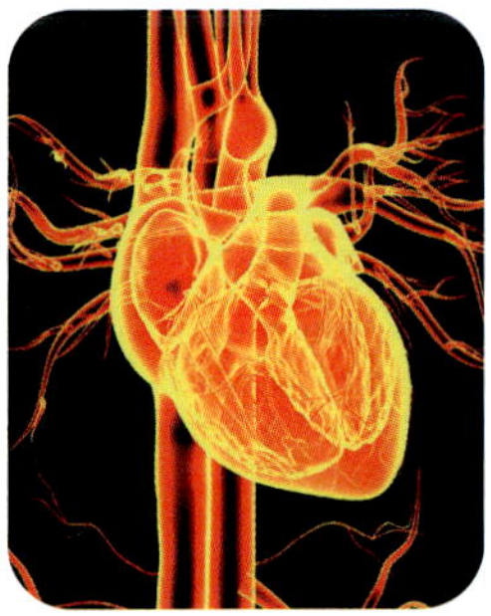

heart (härt) a muscle that pumps blood in your body

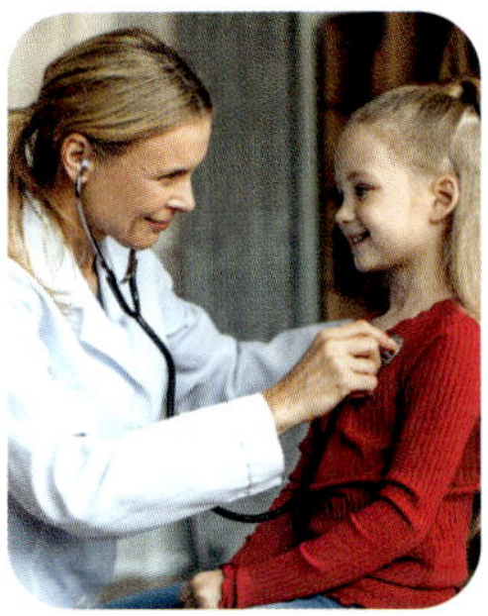

stethoscope (steh-thuh-skōp) a tool doctors use to listen to your heart

Quiz: My Beating Heart

1. Your heart is inside your chest.

   A. Yes B. No

2. Can you feel your heart?

   A. Yes B. No

3. Does your heart beat faster when you run?

   A. Yes B. No

4. Can running and eating good food help your heart?

   A. Yes B. No

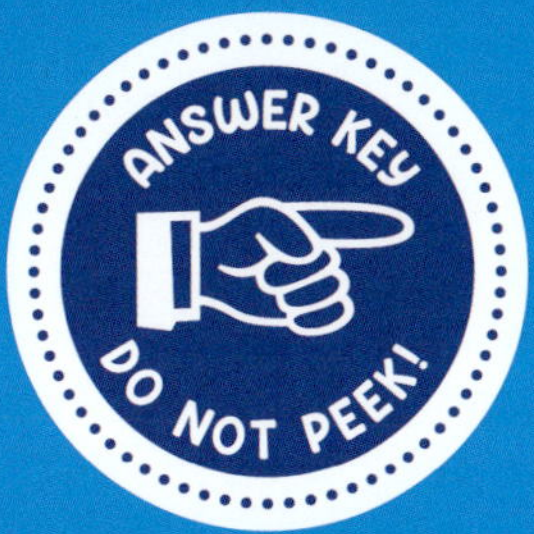

ANSWER KEY:

How many times did you answer yes?

4 Yes: Awesome! You know your heart well.

3 Yes: Great! You learned some new facts.

2 Yes: That's okay! Keep reading.

1 Yes: You're starting to learn. Keep going!

Further Reading

Moore, Dr. Ryan. *Hank the Heart*. Blue Manatee Press, 2020.

Wendt, Jennifer. *My Heart*. Bearport Publishing. 2022.

On the Internet

KidsHealth—Your Heart & Circulatory System

https://kidshealth.org/en/kids/heart.html

This resource describes the heart as a pump that moves blood around the body, providing oxygen and nutrients.

Cool Kid Facts—Human Heart Facts for Kids

https://www.coolkidfacts.com/human-heart-facts-for-kids/

This article offers 10 interesting facts about the heart.

Britannica Kids: Heart

https://kids.britannica.com/kids/article/heart/353235

An explanation of the heart's structure and function, including its role in pumping blood throughout the body.

Index

About the Author

Rachel Daniels is a former elementary school teacher who loves reading and discovering new things. She lives in sunny South Florid with her husband, close to her childre and grandchildren. When she's not reading or writing, she enjoys playing Canasta with friends. Her goal is to make learning exciting and joyful for young readers everywhere.